T

4-Week of Gut Healing

A Science-Based Plan to Repair Your Leaky Gut with Whole Foods and Lifestyle Changes

(Includes 50 Nourishing Recipes to Rebalance Your Microbiome)

Katherine Joe

IMPORTANT NOTE TO READERS

The intention of this book is solely to provide education purpose. The author is not a certified medical professional and this guide should not be used as a replacement for medical advice. If you are experiencing any health issues, diseases, or medical conditions, it is crucial to consult a medical doctor. Prior to engaging in any exercises, nutrition, diets, supplements, or utilizing other health-related information provided/discussed in this book, it is essential to confirm your medical condition by consulting a doctor or healthcare provider for guidance. Haven't executed all efforts, and to the best of the author's knowledge, and belief, the contents of information contains in this book were derived and

Introduction

A healthy gut is the foundation for overall health and wellbeing. However, in our modern world, gut health issues like leaky gut syndrome are becoming increasingly common. Leaky gut occurs when the intestinal lining becomes inflamed and develops microscopic holes that allow undigested foods, toxins, and bacteria to "leak" into the bloodstream. This triggers widespread inflammation and can cause symptoms like bloating, fatigue, skin issues, autoimmune disorders, and more.

The good news is that leaky gut can be healed with the right diet, lifestyle changes, and time. In this 4-week gut healing program, you'll learn the science behind leaky gut and why it matters for your whole body health. Then, you'll be guided through a strategic month-long protocol to remove gut irritants, replace with gut-soothing foods, reinoculate with healthy probiotics, and repair your intestinal lining. With the recipes and lifestyle advice provided, you'll nourish your microbiome and come away with a plan for long-term gut health.

Chapter 1 starts by defining leaky gut syndrome and explaining recent scientific research on how and why it develops. You'll learn how chronic stress, poor diet, medication use, bacterial infections, and other factors can damage the gut lining and tight junctions between intestinal cells. We'll cover how this "leaky" state allows toxins, microbes, and undigested food particles into the bloodstream, triggering widespread inflammation. This can manifest in digestion issues, food sensitivities, autoimmunity, skin conditions, and even mental health disorders. We'll also discuss the profound gut-brain connection and explore how your microbiome impacts your mood, cognition, and nervous system function.

Next, you'll discover why healing your gut is so crucial for overall wellbeing. Optimizing your microbiome diversity leads to better nutrient absorption, reduced inflammation, balanced hormones, improved metabolism, enhanced immunity against pathogens, and more. Feeding your gut the right "fertilizer" in the form of prebiotics has been shown to lessen anxiety and depression as well as improve markers for cardiovascular and metabolic health. With a thriving gut microbiome, your whole body can function at its prime. That's why following the gut healing protocols in this book are so important.

In Chapter 2, we will dive into the comprehensive 4-week plan for repairing leaky gut. Each week focuses on one of the key steps needed to allow your intestinal lining to heal:

Week 1 is about removing gut irritants and inflammatory foods from your diet. These include processed foods, added sugars, conventional dairy, gluten, alcohol, caffeine, and more. I'll provide meal plans and snack ideas that avoid these triggers to calm inflammation and allow your gut to rest and reset.

Week 2 focuses on replacing aggravating foods with gut-soothing, nutrient-dense whole foods. Following an anti-inflammatory, Mediterranean-style diet rich in fiber, healthy fats, and phytonutrients is key. I'll share guidelines on how to shift your diet, including foods and supplements to emphasize like fermented foods, bone broth, collagen, adaptogens, and omega-3s. These provide the building blocks to begin healing your intestinal barrier.

On Week 3, you'll learn how to reinoculate and restore a diversity of beneficial bacteria to your microbiome. Consuming fermented foods daily, taking targeted probiotic supplements, and avoiding unnecessary antibiotics when possible will rebalance your inner ecosystem. This sets the stage for improved nutrient absorption and starting to seal intestinal junctions.

Finally, Week 4 concentrates on providing key nutrients, amino acids, and compounds to further repair and strengthen your intestinal lining. Things like glutamine, zinc carnosine, licorice root, and quercetin help regenerate cells, reduce inflammation, and reinforce the tight junctions between gut cells. Following the protocols in this repair phase can bring longer-lasting gut healing results.

Throughout the month, I'll offer tips on scheduling meals, stocking your healing kitchen, meal prep, and dealing with potential symptoms like die-off from candida overgrowth. With the structure of this 4-week plan and the right motivation, you can overcome leaky gut for good!

In Chapter 3, you'll discover 50 delicious, nourishing recipes to support your gut healing journey. These anti-inflammatory meals, snacks, and drinks are designed to realign your body and microbiome. I've included a diverse array of options so you can find new favorite go-to recipes.

Start your day with antioxidant-rich smoothies and bowls featuring ingredients like berries, spinach, avocado, collagen, turmeric, and adaptogens. Try your hand at ferments like beet kvass, coconut yogurt, and kimchi to boost probiotics. Soothe inflammation with healing soups and salads like turmeric cauliflower soup, Mediterranean chickpea salad, or Thai coconut fish soup.

Main dishes range from sheet pan lemon chicken with roasted veggies to portobello mushroom burgers to salmon with dill and fennel. Each provides a balanced dose of protein, fiber, healthy fats, and micronutrients to satisfy while avoiding gut-aggravating ingredients. You'll also find recipes for gut-friendly sides, sauces, snacks, and desserts like chia pudding, chocolate bark with goji berries, banana muffins, and more.

With this assortment of delicious, nourishing recipes, you'll discover new favorite gut-healing meals and learn cooking techniques that will serve your microbiome for a lifetime. Following the recipes while on your gut repair journey will help speed gut lining healing and rebalance your inner ecosystem.

In Chapter 4, we will explore lifestyle factors outside of diet that are crucial for maintaining long-term gut health. Managing chronic stress through techniques like meditation, yoga, breathwork, and nature time are key, as uncontrolled stress damages gut lining integrity. Establishing consistent sleep habits, with 7-9 hours per night, allows your microbiome and intestines to rejuvenate. Recommended gut-supporting exercises like walking, Pilates, Tai Chi, and others will aid circulation and motility. I'll also share guidance on how to sustain diversity in your microbiome after gut repair through ongoing fermented foods, periodic cleansing, and avoiding unnecessary antibiotic use.

Finally, in the conclusion, we will recap the key steps from the gut healing journey: removing irritants, replacing with soothers, reinoculating microbiome diversity, and repairing intestinal tissues. I'll share inspirational stories from others who have transformed their health through gut healing protocols. You'll come away from this book armed with the knowledge, tools, and motivation to restore gut health, realign your inner ecosystem, and feel your best from the inside out. With the right commitment to support your microbiome, you can overcome leaky gut and achieve vibrant overall wellness.

Chapter 1

Understanding Leaky Gut and Why Your Gut Matters

Your gut is home to over 100 trillion microbes that make up your gut microbiome. This bustling inner ecosystem plays a profound role in your health and wellbeing. When your gut microbiome is balanced, these beneficial bacteria support healthy digestion, nutrient absorption, immunity, metabolism, and more. However, if gut health becomes compromised, it can lead to a condition known as "leaky gut syndrome."

Leaky gut syndrome is on the rise globally, affecting an estimated 50% of people to some degree. It occurs when gaps or openings develop in the intestinal lining, allowing bacteria, toxins, and undigested food particles to leak out from your intestines into the bloodstream. This triggers widespread inflammation and autoimmune reactions. Left untreated, leaky gut can lead to chronic fatigue, food sensitivities, skin conditions, joint pain, autoimmunity, and numerous other issues.

In this chapter, we'll dive into what causes leaky gut syndrome, how it impacts your body and mind, and why healing your microbiome is so crucial for overall wellness. First, let's explore what is happening inside your gut when you have leaky gut.

What is Leaky Gut?

Your small intestine is lined with millions of microscopic folds containing epithelial cells joined together by tight junctions. This inner barrier controls what gets absorbed into your body and what stays in your digestive tract. Within a healthy gut, the tight junctions between epithelial cells are intact, acting as gatekeepers so only fully digested nutrients can pass through the intestinal lining into your bloodstream.

However, when your gut health becomes compromised, these junctions loosen and gaps develop in your intestinal lining. Bacteria, toxins, undigested food particles, and waste products then have free access into the bloodstream. Your immune system sees these compounds as foreign invaders and attacks them, triggering widespread inflammation. Meanwhile, the lining becomes more permeable, continuing the cycle.

Common Causes of Leaky Gut Syndrome

There are many potential causes and contributing factors to developing leaky gut syndrome:

- Chronic stress - Stress hormones like cortisol negatively impact gut barrier integrity and increase intestinal permeability.

- Poor diet - Diets high in processed foods, sugar, saturated fats, and chemical additives promote inflammation.

- Food sensitivities - Gluten, dairy, and other reactive foods commonly trigger leaky gut.

- Medications - Antibiotics, NSAIDs, steroids, antacids and others alter gut flora and hinder cell regeneration.

- Infections - Bacterial, viral, or fungal overgrowths like SIBO, candida, and parasites can damage the gut lining.

- Toxins - Mold, heavy metals, pesticides, and environmental toxins have detrimental effects on intestinal integrity.

- Low stomach acid - Insufficient stomach acid impairs digestion and allows pathogens to proliferate.

- Nutrient deficiencies - Lacking nutrients like zinc, vitamin A, glutamine, or vitamin D inhibit proper cell turnover.

- Autoimmunity - Conditions like celiac, IBS, or lupus have leaky gut involvement.

- Aging - The gut lining can become more porous as we get older.

As you can see, leaky gut has numerous potential causes and risk factors. The more of these you face, the higher your likelihood of developing increased intestinal permeability.

Main Impacts of Leaky Gut Syndrome

Once your intestinal barrier has been breached, the cascade of inflammatory responses that follow can impact your health in myriad ways. Here are some of the main consequences tied to leaky gut syndrome:

Digestive Troubles Since leaky gut permits undigested food particles and bacteria into the bloodstream before proper processing, it commonly manifests through digestive complaints and malabsorption issues. Symptoms like gas, bloating, cramping, constipation, diarrhea, heartburn, and nausea are very common. Nutrient deficiencies may also develop if your damaged gut lining cannot properly break down and uptake nutrients from your food.

Food Sensitivities Leaky gut is linked to developing extra reactivity to foods you previously tolerated. When incompletely broken-down proteins cross your intestinal lining, your body sees them as foreign and makes antibodies against them. You can then develop new intolerances and allergies to those foods. Gluten, dairy, corn, soy, eggs, and nightshades are common culprits.

Inflammation and Pain Chronic low-grade inflammation from leaky gut can manifest as muscle aches, joint pain, headaches, and chronic fatigue. The flood of inflammatory cytokines released in response to gut bacteria and toxins entering your bloodstream leads to this systemic inflammatory response.

Skin Conditions Skin issues like eczema, acne, rashes, and rosacea are often tied to leaky gut. Inflammation from the leaky gut can trigger skin reactions and compound underlying hormonal imbalances. Healing your gut is foundational for clearing inflammatory skin disorders.

Autoimmunity

Intestinal permeability is linked to development of autoimmune diseases like Hashimoto's hypothyroidism, rheumatoid arthritis, lupus, multiple sclerosis, and more. When foreign invaders breach the gut lining, it confuses your immune system and makes it more prone to attacking your own tissues.

Mood Disorders Leaky gut allows compounds like lipopolysaccharides to enter your bloodstream and travel to your brain, provoking neuroinflammation that can manifest as anxiety, brain fog, and depression. Healing your gut may alleviate mental health disorders.

As you can see, the downstream effects of leaky gut syndrome can impact your life in countless ways. Let's now discuss why having optimal gut health matters beyond just addressing leaky gut.

Why Your Gut Matters

We've explored the consequences of an unhealthy, permeable gut, but what are the upsides of supporting optimal gut function? As the gatekeeper of what enters your body from the outside world, your GI system plays a monumental role in your overall health and longevity. Here's an overview of the key benefits of prioritizing gut health:

Nutrient Absorption A healthy intestinal villi is covered with microvilli that assimilate nutrients from food and transport them into your bloodstream. With leaky gut, your cell turnover may be impaired and lead to fewer microvilli, poor digestion of foods, and malnutrition. Promoting a healthy gut optimizes your ability to absorb essential nutrients.

Immune Function Over 70% of your immune system resides in and around your GI tract. The gut-associated lymphoid tissue (GALT) releases antibodies, antimicrobial compounds, and more to protect against invading pathogens. When your gut lining is damaged, it allows more bacteria in and taxes your immune resources.

Detoxifying your Gut helps eliminate toxins like pesticides, heavy metals, and mold metabolites. Intestinal cells help modify toxin molecules to make them easier to excrete. With leaky gut, toxins may overwhelm your detox processes.

Inflammation Reduction A thriving gut microbiome helps control inflammatory pathways in the body by reducing inflammatory cytokines and increasing regulatory T cells. Leaky gut allows inflammatory compounds into the blood, heightening inflammation.

Metabolic Regulation Your gut microbiome impacts how well you process carbs and fats, extract energy from food, and maintain healthy blood sugar regulation. An unhealthy gut can contribute to insulin resistance, weight gain, and diabetes.

Hormone Balance Your gut helps regulate major hormonal pathways including thyroid hormone, estrogen, testosterone, melatonin, and stress hormones. Leaky gut can exacerbate hormone deficiencies or excesses.

Mood and Cognition Your gut microbiome produces key neurotransmitters like serotonin, GABA, and acetylcholine that communicate with your brain via the gut-brain axis. An unhealthy microbiome balance can affect your mood, mental health, and brain function.

As you can see, ensuring your gut is healthy not only resolves immediate digestive issues, but also has far-reaching benefits for your whole body down to your cellular and metabolic processes. That's why adopting the gut healing diet and lifestyle protocols covered in this book are so vital.

The Gut-Brain Connection

Now that we've covered the basics of leaky gut causes and impacts, let's dive deeper into one of the most fascinating gut-related topics: the gut-brain axis. This explores the profound bidirectional communication network between your gastrointestinal tract and your brain.

Your gut and brain are continuously sending signals back and forth via your nervous system, immune system, and endocrine system. As covered earlier, when your intestinal lining is inflamed and permeable, it allows pro-inflammatory compounds into your bloodstream that can travel to your brain and impact mood and cognition.

But your brain can also send signals that directly impact your gut function. For example, chronic stress produces cortisol and inflammatory biomarkers that can damage your intestinal barrier integrity. The brain and gut are intimately interconnected.

Your gut microbiome may also impact your brain function in numerous ways, including:

- Producing neurotransmitters like serotonin, dopamine, and GABA

- Communicating with the vagus nerve, a superhighway between the gut and brain

- Regulating immune-inflammatory pathways tied to mental health disorders

- Influencing gene expression related to learning, memory, and mood

- Providing key nutrients for brain cell growth and myelin sheath integrity

Fascinating new research is also uncovering how your microbiome may influence brain structure and development. Germ-free mice raised without any gut microbes have shown differences in areas like memory, anxiety, depression, and motor control compared to mice with normal gut flora.

In humans, one study found that infants with more diverse gut bacteria by 1 month old had more robust brain growth and maturation in regions tied to executive function, emotional processing, and memory compared to infants with less diverse microbiomes. Your gut bacteria diversity and overall microbiome health may predict key aspects of future brain structure!

Other studies show that dysbiosis in gut flora is tied to brain fog, anxiety, depression, OCD, bipolar disorder, autism spectrum disorders, and even neurodegenerative diseases like Alzheimer's and Parkinson's. While research is still ongoing in humans, evidence points to the importance of your gut health for both short-term cognitive function and long-term brain integrity.

So in addition to all the digestive and metabolic benefits, optimizing your gut microbiome may also help reduce inflammation in your brain, elevate your mood, boost focus and concentration, and support neurological resilience. Pretty remarkable for an ecosystem of tiny microbes!

Key Takeaways:

In this chapter, we covered what exactly leaky gut syndrome is, what causes it, and how it can impact your physical and mental health in significant ways. We also discussed the immense importance of your gastrointestinal system for nutrient absorption, hormone regulation, immunity, detoxification, metabolism, and even brain function.

Some key takeaways include:

- Leaky gut occurs when gaps develop in your intestinal barrier allowing bacteria, toxins, and undigested food particles to leak from your gut into the bloodstream.

- Contributors include chronic stress, food sensitivities, infections, medications, poor diet, aging, and autoimmunity.

- Leaky gut can manifest in issues like IBS, food intolerances, arthritis, skin conditions, autoimmunity, inflammation, and mental health disorders.

- Supporting gut health optimizes nutrition, reduces inflammation, balances hormones, aids detoxification, regulates metabolism, and may enhance brain function.

- Your gut microbiome communicates with your brain via the gut-brain axis, impacting mental health, cognition, and even neurological development.

- Healing your leaky gut and cultivating a thriving microbiome should be a top wellness goal!

Now that you understand why your gut health matters so profoundly, let's move on to Chapter 2 which will outline the comprehensive gut healing protocols covered in this program. Get ready to learn exactly what to remove, replace, reinoculate, and repair to transform your microbiome and gut health starting today!

Chapter 2

The 4-Week Plan to Heal Leaky Gut

In the previous chapter, we explored what leaky gut is, what causes it, and how it impacts overall health. Now we'll dive into the 4-week gut healing plan to start repairing your intestinal barrier and cultivating a thriving inner ecosystem.

Each week of the program focuses on one of the key steps needed to allow your gut lining to heal:

Week 1 - Remove gut irritants and inflammatory triggers

Week 2 - Replace with gut-soothing foods/supplements

Week 3 - Reinoculate with beneficial bacteria

Week 4 - Repair the gut lining.

Removing inflammatory and irritating foods gives your system a rest. Replacing with nourishing foods and supplements provides the building blocks to heal. Reinoculating restores balanced gut flora for improved immunity and function. Repairing seals the intestinal junctions and aids tissue regeneration.

When done in this sequential order, you can start reversing leaky gut damage and seeing improvements in symptoms. Let's explore each of the weekly protocols in detail.

Week 1: Remove

The first week of your gut healing journey focuses on removing inflammatory foods, gut irritants, and anything else that may compromise your intestinal barrier. This removal process gives your GI tract a chance to calm inflammation and reset.

Here are the main elements to remove during Week 1:

- **Eliminate inflammatory foods -** These include refined sugars, processed grains, conventional dairy, factory-farmed meat, fried foods, alcohol, and artificial additives. An anti-inflammatory, whole food Mediterranean-style diet is ideal.

- **Remove gut irritants -** The main irritants to avoid are gluten, soy, corn, eggs, and nightshades. If you have autoimmunity, also remove grains and legumes.

- **Avoid foods you're sensitive to -** If you experience symptoms like bloating, fatigue, or brain fog after eating certain foods, remove those from your diet for now to allow gut recovery. Common culprits include dairy, gluten, yeast, nuts, eggs, and nightshades.

- **Remove Gut-disrupting Medications -** Avoid unnecessary use of NSAIDs, antibiotics, antacids, and steroids which can impair gut function. Check with your doctor before stopping prescription medications.

- **Eliminate Gut-damaging behaviors -** Reduce alcohol, tobacco, unnecessary antibiotics, high-intensity exercise, and chronic stress during your gut healing journey as these negatively impact your microbiome.

- **Get Extra Sleep -** Aim for 8-9 hours per night to allow your gut time to rest and repair. Sleep is crucial for balancing hormones, lowering inflammation, and healing a leaky gut.

As you remove inflammatory foods and irritants, focus your diet on easy-to-digest foods like bone broth, soups, smoothies, and steamed vegetables which give your GI tract ample nutrients while allowing it to rest. Be sure to stay hydrated with filtered water throughout the day. Herbal teas like chamomile, mint, and ginger are very soothing.

Week 1 Meal Ideas:

— **Breakfast:** Scrambled eggs with spinach, avocado toast, chia pudding, smoothie with banana, blueberries, and collagen powder

— **Lunch:** Vegetable soup, large salad with chicken or salmon and olive oil based dressing

— **Dinner:** Baked white fish with roasted Brussels sprouts and sweet potato, coconut curry chicken soup or stew

— **Snacks:** Fresh berries, raw carrots and hummus, bulletproof coffee, trail mix with nuts and seeds

The first 7 days removing gut irritants allows inflammation levels to decrease so your intestinal lining can start healing in Week 2. Let's explore what to add in during the replace phase.

Week 2: Replace

In Week 2 of your gut healing plan, the focus shifts to replacing inflammatory foods with nourishing ingredients that provide the nutrients your gut needs to repair and regenerate. Emphasize these gut-healing superfoods:

- **Bone broth** - Glycine and proline in broth help heal your intestinal barrier. Sip 1-2 cups per day.

- **Wild fish** - Omega-3 fats in salmon, mackerel, sardines, and anchovies reduce inflammation. Eat 2-3 times per week.

- **Fermented foods** - Sauerkraut, kimchi, kefir, and kombucha contain probiotics to improve microbial balance.

- **Leafy greens** - Spinach, kale, chard, and lettuces provide anti-inflammatory phytonutrients, chlorophyll, and fiber.

- **Pastured eggs** - Rich in 18 amino acids, eggs nourish your gut lining to help repair damaged tissue.

- **Healthy fats** - Coconut oil, ghee, olive oil, avocado oil, nuts, seeds, and their butters provide anti-inflammatory fats.

- **Herbal teas** - Licorice, marshmallow root, ginger, and chamomile tea help soothe and heal your gut lining.

In addition to diet, several gut-healing supplements are beneficial during your replace phase:

- **L-Glutamine powder** - This amino acid helps regenerate intestinal cells and seal leaky gut. Take 5-10 grams daily.

- **Collagen peptides** - Collagens types I, III, V, and X repair damaged intestinal tissue and strengthen your gut barrier. Have 1-2 scoops daily.

- **Adaptogens** - Herbs like ashwagandha, holy basil, and ginseng help your body adapt to stress, a gut irritant. Take as directed.

- **Quercetin** - This antioxidant flavonoid helps reduce inflammation and histamine responses in the gut. Take 500-1000 mg daily with meals.

- **Aloe vera juice** - The polysaccharides in aloe help heal the gut lining and reduce intestinal permeability. Drink 2 oz. daily.

When replacing irritants with gut-soothing foods and supplements, you provide your body the building blocks it needs to start mending

your intestinal barrier and reducing
inflammation.

Week 2 Meal Replacement Ideas:

— **Breakfast:** Vegetable omelet with greens, collagen coffee or smoothie, chia porridge

— **Lunch:** Coconut curry chicken or salmon over cauliflower rice, lentil and veggie soup

— **Dinner:** Grass-fed beef stir fry with cabbage, chicken veggie coconut curry, baked wild salmon

— **Snacks:** Carrot sticks, coconut yogurt with berries, boiled eggs, seed crackers with almond butter

Stick with the replace phase for 7 days while you continue avoiding dietary triggers. Then we'll move to reinoculating your gut microbiome.

Week 3: Reinoculate

In Week 3 of your gut healing plan, the focus shifts to reinoculating your microbiome with beneficial strains of bacteria to repopulate a diversity of flora.

A damaged gut is often overrun with inflammatory species like E. coli, Clostridium difficile, Staphylococcus aureus, and Candida. You need to tip the scales back towards more favorable bugs like Lactobacillus, Bifidobacterium, Akkermansia, and Faecalibacterium prausnitzii.

Here are effective ways to reinoculate your gut's beneficial bacteria:

- Take a multi-strain probiotic supplement with at least 30 billion CFUs from reputable brands. Look for diversity in Lactobacillus, Bifidobacterium, and Saccharomyces strains.

- Consume traditionally fermented foods like sauerkraut, pickles, kefir, kimchi, kombucha, and yogurt. Have 1-2 servings daily. Make sure they contain live cultures.

- Drink bone broth, which contains glycosaminoglycans that act as prebiotics to feed good gut flora. Aim for 1-2 cups per day.

- Eat prebiotic fibers like acacia gum, psyllium husk, dandelion greens, garlic, banana, onion, asparagus, and artichokes which provide "fertilizer" for probiotics.

- Consider taking a spore-based probiotic like Megasporebiotic that gets deep into your intestines to expand flora diversity.

- Avoid unnecessary antibiotics which wipe out good flora. Only take when absolutely needed for infections. Always follow with probiotics.

Reinoculating with a diverse array of microbes trains your immune system to recognize commensal bacteria and improves intestinal barrier function. Don't forget to continue avoiding irritating foods and emphasizing gut-healing nutrition during Week 3.

Week 3 Meal Reinoculation Ideas:

— **Breakfast:** Kefir smoothie with collagen, berries and spinach OR miso soup with seaweed and tofu

— **Lunch:** Kombucha, sauerkraut, carrot ginger soup with coconut milk

— **Dinner:** Coconut curry chicken with cauliflower rice OR grass-fed beef chili with sweet potato

— **Snacks:** Handful of blueberries, half an avocado with sunflower seeds, cultured veggies, banana with almond or cashew butter

Continue reinoculating your gut flora for 7 days before moving to the final repair phase. This allows time for your microbiome balance to improve before sealing the leaks.

Week 4: Repair

In the final phase of your gut healing journey, we shift the focus to repairing and sealing your intestinal barrier by providing key amino acids, antioxidants, and nutrients.

Some of the top gut-repairing nutrients to emphasize now are:

- **L-Glutamine:** This versatile amino acid regenerates intestinal cells and promotes production of tight junction proteins between gut cells. Take 10-30 grams daily.

- **Zinc carnosine:** Zinc helps heal your intestinal lining while L-carnosine combats leaky gut-induced inflammation. Take 75-200 mg, twice daily.

- **Aloe vera:** The polysaccharides in aloe help heal intestinal membranes, reduce inflammation, and decrease permeability. Drink 2 oz. twice daily.

- **Slippery elm:** The mucilage in slippery elm helps coat and soothe your gut lining to aid in repair. Take 400 mg, 2-3x daily.

- **Butyrate:** This short-chain fatty acid nourishes colon cells, improves tight junctions, and reduces intestinal inflammation. Take 1,500 mg daily.

- **Marshmallow root:** Marshmallow contains mucilage that protects and heals the gut lining. Take 400 mg, 2-3x daily.

- **DGL licorice:** The glycyrrhizin in DGL licorice combats leaky gut-induced inflammation in the intestines. Chew 350-1000 mg tablets, as needed.

In addition to supplements, emphasize natural foods high in these repairing nutrients like bone broth, grass-fed gelatin, spirulina, avocado, cabbage, and snap peas.

Continue avoiding inflammatory and harsh foods. Keep reinoculating with probiotics and fermented foods while providing plenty of antioxidants from your meals like berries, dark leafy greens, carrots, and herbs like turmeric.

Week 4 Meal Repair Ideas:

— **Breakfast:** Eggs with veggies and sprouted grain toast OR Berry coconut smoothie with collagen

— **Lunch:** Buffalo chicken lettuce wraps with carrots and celery OR Lentil veggie soup

— **Dinner:** Sheet pan salmon with Brussels sprouts and butternut squash OR Ground turkey lettuce tacos

— **Snacks:** Roasted chickpeas, half an avocado with sunflower seeds, cucumber slices, zucchini muffins

Make it through the entire 4 weeks avoiding reactive foods, emphasizing gut-soothers, reinoculating with probiotics, and focusing on key repairing nutrients. By the end, your gut should be well on its way towards healing!

Additional Gut Healing Tips

Here are some additional tips to further support your gut healing journey:

- Manage stress with meditation, deep breathing, yoga, nature time, or other relaxing activities to avoid cortisol-induced intestinal damage.

- Consider trying bone broth fasting, a gentle cleanse, or intermittent fasting periodically to give your digestion a rest.

- Support colon motility through exercise, magnesium, antioxidants, and probiotics to avoid constipation and help sweep toxins out.

- Rotate your diet or try elimination protocols like Paleo or AIP if reacting to multiple foods to help identify triggers.

- Come off gut-damaging medications like antacids, antibiotics or NSAIDs under medical supervision if possible.

- Address underlying infections through functional testing and appropriate antimicrobial or antiparasitic protocols.

- Consider digestive enzymes or betaine HCl supplements if low stomach acid is an issue limiting your nutrient absorption.

- Check for hidden sources of gluten, soy, eggs or dairy if reacting to those. Be meticulous.

- Reduce toxin exposure by choosing organic produce, natural body products, an air purifier, and filtering your water,

- Monitor symptoms and take notes on which therapies help you feel better or worse to refine your protocol.

The more diligent you can be at avoiding reactive foods, emphasizing gut healers, cultivating healthy flora, and providing repair nutrients, the quicker you'll see results. Be patient, as significant gut healing often takes months. But stick with it, and you can overcome leaky gut!

Key Takeaways:

Those are the specifics of the 4-week gut healing plan focused on removing, replacing, reinoculating, and repairing your microbiome and intestinal barrier. Here are some key takeaways:

- Follow the 4-step protocol in sequence for 1 week each to allow gut lining repair.

- Remove inflammatory foods and gut irritants during Week 1. Emphasize easy-to-digest foods.

- Replace with gut nourishing foods and supplements like collagen, glutamine, adaptogens in Week 2.

- Reinoculate your microbial diversity through probiotics and fermented foods in Week 3.

- Week 4 seals your intestinal lining using nutrients like glutamine, zinc, licorice, and aloe vera.

- Support each phase with ample filtered water, herbal teas, healing spices, stress-relieving activities, and 8+ hours of sleep nightly.

Your digestive system is home to your second brain - your enteric nervous system. Healing your gut truly allows the rest of your body and mind to heal! Now that you understand the comprehensive 4-step protocol, let's dive into the delicious gut-healing recipes in Chapter 3 next.

Chapter 3

50 Nourishing Recipes to Support Your Gut Health Journey

Now that you understand the science behind healing leaky gut and the 4-week protocol, let's explore how to put that into action in your kitchen! In this chapter, we'll cover 50 delicious anti-inflammatory recipes using gut-soothing ingredients to help you along your gut healing journey.

These recipes span gut-friendly breakfasts, salads and soups, prebiotic-rich main dishes, fermented foods and drinks, and healing elixirs. You'll find options that fit nicely within the 4-week gut healing plan outlined in Chapter 2.

The ingredients called for in these recipes were specially selected to calm inflammation, soothe your digestive system, provide nutrients that regenerate gut tissue, expand beneficial microbes, and remove irritating compounds. Cooking and eating your way through these recipes will help speed gut recovery.

A. Anti-Inflammatory Breakfasts

Let's start the day off right with some nourishing breakfast options that avoid common gut aggravators like gluten grains, dairy, and sugar while emphasizing phytonutrients, collagen, healthy fats, and fiber:

1. **Chia Pudding -** Combine chia seeds, unsweetened coconut milk or almond milk, collagen peptides, cinnamon, and your choice of berries in a mason jar. Refrigerate overnight. The chia provides omega-3 fats and gel for intestinal barrier protection.

2. **Poached Eggs over Greens -** Lightly sauté some Swiss chard, spinach, or kale in olive oil or ghee. Add herbs like basil, dill, or parsley. Top with 1-2 poached or boiled pastured eggs. The eggs provide protein, healthy fats, and bioavailable nutrients to nourish your gut.

3. **Bone Broth Power Smoothie -** Blend collagen powder, frozen berries, banana, avocado, almond milk, ginger, turmeric, and a dash of nutmeg with 1 cup warm bone broth for a smoothie containing amino acids and nutrients to restore gut health. The collagen in particular aids in intestinal healing.

4. **Mushroom and Asparagus Frittata -** Whisk together a dozen eggs with some cream or coconut milk. Add diced

mushrooms, asparagus, spinach, onions, garlic, salt, and pepper and pour into a greased baking dish. Bake at 350F for 20-25 minutes. Mushrooms contain polysaccharides that enhance immune function.

5. **Tigernut Granola Parfait** - In a jar layer nuts, seeds, unsweetened coconut, cinnamon tigernut granola with Greek yogurt or coconut yogurt and berries. Tigernuts provide prebiotic fiber to feed microbiome diversity.

6. **Carrot, Turmeric and Ginger Juice** - Juice carrots, lemon, fresh turmeric and ginger for an anti-inflammatory and cleansing drink.

7. **Coconut Yogurt Parfait -** Layer coconut yogurt with berries, bee pollen, hemp seeds, cinnamon and RAW honey.

8. **Zucchini Muffins -** Make grain-free muffins with almond flour, zucchini, applesauce, cinnamon, baking powder, eggs, vanilla and chocolate chips

9. **Vegetable Scramble -** Lightly cook spinach, mushrooms, onions and tomatoes in coconut oil. Add beaten eggs and scramble

10. **Pineapple Ginger Sorbet -** Blend frozen pineapple, ginger powder, lemon juice and coconut cream for a dairy-free anti-inflammatory "sorbet".

These anti-inflammatory breakfasts avoid common gut irritants while providing nutrients to seal and soothe your intestinal barrier. Great way to start your day on the road to gut wellness!

B. Gut-Soothing Soups and Salads

Warm brothy soups and crisp salads are very soothing for your digestion and provide an easy way to emphasize gut-healing foods. Try these recipes:

11. **Chicken Zoodle Soup -** Spiralize zucchini into noodles and add to a pot with homemade bone broth, cooked shredded chicken, carrots, celery, onion, garlic, basil, oregano, salt and pepper. Let simmer 5-10 minutes. The amino acids in bone broth heal and seal your gut lining.

12. **Turmeric Lentil Stew -** In a soup pot sauté onions, garlic, celery, and carrots. Add broth, green lentils, kale, sweet

potato, turmeric, cumin, coriander, salt, and pepper. Simmer until lentils are tender, about 25-30 minutes. The spices provide anti-inflammatory compounds while lentils feed your gut flora.

13. **Mediterranean Tuna Salad** - Mix together canned tuna, diced cucumber, bell pepper, cherry tomatoes, Kalamata olives, olive oil, lemon juice, parsley, mint, and onion. Serve on a bed of greens. The olive oil, herbs, and vegetables provide anti-inflammatory phytonutrients to heal your gut.

14. **Kimchi Noodle Jar** - Layer a mason jar with kimchi, cooked rice noodles, carrot ribbons, sliced mushrooms, baby bok choy, basil, cilantro, sesame oil, soy sauce, Sriracha, and sesame seeds. The

fermented kimchi provides probiotics to balance your gut flora.

15. **Cabbage Detox Salad** – Shred green and purple cabbage and carrots and toss with lemon juice, apple cider vinegar, olive oil, parsley, cilantro, salt and pepper. Top with sunflower seeds. Cabbage is very soothing for your digestive lining.

16. **Rosemary and Thyme Roasted Chicken** - Roast a whole chicken rubbed with fresh rosemary, thyme, garlic, lemon and olive oil. Serve with roasted vegetables

17. **Coconut Curry Soup** - Cook cauliflower, sweet potato and carrots in coconut milk with curry powder, ginger and collagen for a nourishing soup.

18. **Chicken Vegetable Soup -** Simmer chicken, carrots, celery, onions, mushrooms, garlic, thyme, sea salt and rice noodles in bone broth for a complete gut-soothing meal.

19. **Tuna Salad Lettuce Wraps -** Mix tuna with avocado mayo, celery, onion and herbs. Serve in butter lettuce leaves.

20. **Roasted Root Vegetables -** Toss carrots, sweet potatoes, beets, parsnips and onions with avocado oil and roast at 400F until tender and caramelized.

21. **Mediterranean Tuna Salad -** Mix tuna, artichoke hearts, olives, cucumber, red bell pepper, olive oil, lemon, garlic, dill, parsley.

22. **Cucumber Dill Salad -** Toss cucumbers, red onion and dill with apple cider vinegar, olive oil and sea salt. Enjoy the probiotic benefits of vinegars.

23. **Guacamole -** Mash avocado with lime juice, onion, tomato, cilantro and sea salt for a quick probiotic and fiber-rich snack.

These soups and salads provide fiber, phytonutrients, fermented probiotics, and broth to reduce intestinal inflammation while expanding gut flora diversity.

C. Main Dishes Packed with Prebiotics

Get creative with gut-friendly main dishes centered on prebiotic fibers that act as "fertilizer" for the beneficial microbes in your microbiome:

24. **Salmon Sheet Pan Dinner** – Roast wild salmon alongside Brussels sprouts, sweet potato, red onion, garlic, and olive oil on a baking sheet in the oven at 400F for 15-20 minutes. The prebiotic fiber in the sprouts will enhance the microbiome benefits of the omega-3 rich salmon.

25. **Chicken and Vegetable Stir Fry** – Sauté onions, carrots, broccoli, snow peas, mushrooms, garlic, ginger, and tamari or coconut aminos. Add cooked chicken, sesame oil, rice vinegar, and crushed red pepper and toss. Serve over cauliflower rice. Mushrooms and onion contain prebiotic oligosaccharides.

26. **Zucchini Lasagna** – Make lasagna layers using long slices of zucchini instead of pasta, along with tomato sauce, basil,

cooked ground turkey or beef, mushrooms, spinach, artichokes, ricotta or goat cheese, and marinara sauce. The zucchini provides gut-soothing cucurbitacins.

27. **Cassava Flour Flatbreads** – Mix cassava flour, olive oil, baking powder, salt and water into a dough. Roll out and pan fry 3-5 minutes per side. Top with avocado, microgreens, smoked salmon, and lemon juice. Cassava contains the prebiotic fiber inulin which is well-tolerated.

28. **Grass-fed Beef Chili** – Brown grass-fed ground beef with onions, peppers, and garlic. Add tomato sauce, carrots, zucchini, chili seasoning, bone broth, and black beans. Simmer 20 minutes. Top with avocado, green onion, and cilantro.

The resistant starch in beans feeds gut flora.

29.Salmon Cakes - Make patties with canned salmon, almond flour, dill, garlic, eggs, parsley and old bay seasoning. Pan fry in coconut oil.

30.Gut-Healing Bone Broth - Simmer beef or chicken bones with vegetables, apple cider vinegar and herbs for at least 12-24 hours to extract gut-soothing amino acids.

31.Wild Blueberry Gelatin - Make sugar-free gelatin with wild blueberry juice and dissolve in heated bone broth instead of water for added amino acid benefits.

Packing your meals with prebiotic fibers helps nourish the beneficial microbes that aid digestion, improve immunity, and strengthen your intestinal barrier against leaky gut development.

D. Probiotic-Boosting Fermented Foods and Drinks

Naturally fermented foods are brimming with beneficial bacteria that help repopulate a diversity of flora in your microbiome. Try including these recipes:

32. **Kefir Smoothie –** Blend together kefir, frozen berries, banana, spinach or kale, ground flaxseed, cinnamon, and nut butter for a smoothie containing probiotics to balance your inner ecosystem.

33. **Kombucha Float –** Pour a glass of ginger-flavored kombucha and add a

scoop of coconut ice cream or gelato on top. The effervescent bubbles plus live probiotic cultures make a gut-healing treat.

34. **Cultured Salsa –** Blend chopped tomatoes, onion, peppers, lime juice, cilantro, and avocado with a dollop of coconut milk kefir or yogurt. Use as a salsa with flax crackers or cucumber slices.

35. **Beet Kvass –** Chop and blend beets with garlic, ginger, salt, and water. Allow to ferment 2-3 days. Strain and drink the juice. Beets have natural probiotic benefits.

36. **Homemade Yogurt -** Heat milk on the stove just until steaming. Cool to 110F and add a few spoonfuls of a probiotic

yogurt starter. Allow to ferment overnight. Transfer to the fridge by morning. Use this yogurt in smoothies, parfaits, curry sauces, and more to add beneficial bacteria to your diet.

37. Fennel Detox Tea - Steep fennel seeds in hot water for an anti-inflammatory tea that also aids digestion.

38. Ginger Peach Smoothie - Blend frozen peaches, ginger, vanilla Greek yogurt, collagen and almond milk for a cream probiotic smoothie.

Sipping fermented drinks like kvass and kombucha as well as eating cultured foods like yogurt, kefir, and sauerkraut gives your gut live strains of bacteria that help rebalance your microbiome and improve the integrity of your intestinal barrier.

E. Herbal Teas and Healing Elixirs

Sipping on comforting herbal teas can help provide antioxidants and soothing compounds to reduce intestinal inflammation in leaky gut:

39. **Slippery Elm Tea -** Steep slippery elm bark in hot water for 10+ minutes to release the gut-coating mucilage that protects and repairs your intestinal lining. Sweeten with a bit of maple syrup or raw honey if desired.

40. **Marshmallow Root Tea –** Just like slippery elm, marshmallow root contains healing mucilage when steeped in hot water. Drink 1-2 cups per day on an empty stomach to coat and soothe your digestive tract.

41. **Ginger Lemon Tea –** Fresh grated ginger root steeped in hot water with

lemon juice and raw honey provides anti-inflammatory phenols to help heal your gut lining.

42. **Peppermint Tea –** The volatile oils in peppermint are very soothing for digestion and calming gut spasms or discomfort. Steep fresh or dried leaves in hot water 5-7 minutes.

43. **Turmeric Golden Milk -** Combine turmeric powder, grated ginger, cinnamon, cardamom, vanilla, and nutmeg in warm coconut or almond milk sweetened with honey. Turmeric contains curcumin which can help heal ulcers in your intestinal lining.

44. Cardamom Hot Chocolate - Heat coconut milk with cacao powder,

cinnamon, nutmeg and cardamom for a gut-soothing dairy-free hot chocolate.

45. Pear Cranberry Crisp - Bake sliced pears and cranberries topped with a mix of almonds, oats, coconut, cinnamon, nutmeg, maple syrup and coconut oil.

Sipping these herbal teas between meals gives your GI tract beneficial plant compounds while delivering hydration to support every stage of your gut healing regimen.

F. Gut-Soothing Desserts and Snacks

You can still satisfy sweet cravings and enjoy tasty snacks while nourishing your gut:

46. **Berry Gelatin Parfait –** Dissolve grass-fed collagen peptides into heated bone broth and pour into molds with your

choice of berries. Chill to create gut-healing protein pudding.

47. **Avocado Chocolate Pudding** – Blend avocado, cacao powder, and your choice of milk or yogurt for a decadent, anti-inflammatory chocolate mousse-like treat.

48. **Chewy Granola Bars -** Mix oats, seeds, nuts, coconut, nut butter, cinnamon, vanilla, and just a touch of maple syrup. Press into a parchment-lined dish and bake 25 minutes at 375F. Allow to cool and slice into bars for a satisfying snack containing prebiotics.

49. **Gingerbread Smoothie** – Blend a frozen banana, avocado, almond milk, collagen peptides, cinnamon, ginger, nutmeg, cloves, and vanilla for a smoothie that

tastes like a gingerbread cookie but soothes your gut.

50. **Carrot Cake Bites –** Mix grated carrots, almond flour, applesauce, cinnamon, allspice, ginger, coconut oil, maple syrup, and vanilla extract. Form into bite-sized balls and bake 10-15 minutes at 350F. Makes a gut-friendly mini "cake" high in carotenoids.

Enjoying these nourishing snacks keeps your microbiome and intestinal barrier happy.

Key Takeaways:

There you have 50 amazing recipes spanning smoothies, soups, salads, main dishes, fermented foods, elixirs, desserts, and more to include in your 4-week gut healing protocol and continue emphasizing until leaky gut is resolved.

Some key points about these recipes:

- They emphasize easy-to-digest yet nourishing ingredients shown clinically to heal leaky gut like collagen, bone broth, healthy fats, herbs, and prebiotics.

- They avoid common gut irritants like gluten, dairy, processed foods, sugars, and excessive fiber.

- They provide anti-inflammatory compounds from plants to soothe an inflamed intestinal lining.

- Fermented foods and collagen support probiotics and tissue regeneration.

- Options make following an elimination diet or low FODMAP diet doable.

- Variety covers all meals and snacks so gut healing can become a lifestyle.

Eating this way consistently removes sources of irritation, provides nutrients that regenerate your intestinal barrier, expands microbiome diversity, and resolves inflammation. Combined with the 4-week gut healing protocols from Chapter 2, you now have all the tools needed to conquer leaky gut for good!

Chapter 4

Optimizing Your Lifestyle for Long-Term Gut Health

In the previous chapters, we covered dietary protocols and delicious recipes to help you heal leaky gut. However, certain lifestyle factors outside of nutrition can also have a big impact on balancing your microbiome and maintaining a healthy gut lining long-term.

In this chapter, we'll explore how managing stress, prioritizing sleep, engaging in gut-supportive exercises, and sustaining microbiome diversity after gut healing protocols are key for preserving your hard-won gut health gains. Let's look at each of these crucial lifestyle components.

Managing Stress for Optimal Gut Wellbeing

Stress, especially when chronic, can wreak havoc on your gastrointestinal function. Stress triggers your sympathetic nervous system, activating your fight-or-flight response. This causes release of stress hormones like cortisol and adrenaline which have many detrimental effects:

- Alters gut motility and transit time, contributing to either constipation or diarrhea

- Decreases blood flow and oxygenation to the GI tract

- Reduces nutrient absorption and alters microbial populations

- Compromises intestinal barrier integrity, promoting leaky gut

81

- Shifts immune activity away from the gut, allowing pathogens to proliferate

- Triggers inflammation and oxidative stress in the intestinal lining

Left unchecked, these stress-induced changes impair digestion, perpetuate leaky gut, and allow harmful bacteria and toxins into circulation. This sparks widespread inflammation that can worsen mood disorders, pain levels, and various health conditions.

Managing your stress levels through lifestyle techniques is essential for maintaining optimal gut health. Here are some effective stress relief strategies:

- Daily meditation or breathwork practices - Meditating activates the parasympathetic "rest and digest" system, reversing the effects of stress. Just 5-10 minutes per day can impart significant benefits.

- Yoga and Tai Chi - Gentle movement paired with focused breathing elicits deep relaxation while stimulating circulation and motility.

- Nature time and forest bathing - Spending time outdoors surrounded by nature provides phytoncides from plants that reduce inflammation and cortisol levels.

- Massage, acupuncture, reflexology - Hands-on modalities help release stored tension, reduce blood pressure, and relax the nervous system.

- Float therapy - Floating effortlessly in a sensory deprivation pod induces the deepest state of relaxation, allowing gut tissues to regenerate.

- Gratitude journaling - Focusing on blessings counteracts the brain's negativity bias, lowering stress-induced inflammation.

- Creative hobbies - Pursuits like art, music, dance, and crafts engross your mind, providing a respite from worrying thoughts.

- Laughing and play - Laughter is proven to decrease cortisol, relieve anxiety, improve oxygenation, and support healthy gut motility.

By engaging in relaxing activities every day, especially those involving deep breathing, you counteract the physical effects of stress and allow your GI system to function optimally.

Protect your gut health by making stress management a priority.

The Importance of Adequate Sleep for Gut Health

In addition to managing stress levels, getting sufficient high-quality sleep is crucial for maintaining a healthy gut microbiome and intestinal barrier function. While you sleep, your body produces melatonin, an antioxidant that suppresses inflammation while stimulating protective compounds and stem cells that regenerate the intestinal lining. Sleep is also when your gut microbial profile shifts towards more favorable constituents like Bifidobacterium and Lactobacillus.

Insufficient or disrupted sleep negatively affects your gut in several ways:

- Increases intestinal permeability and low-grade inflammation

- Alters tight junction proteins that seal the intestinal barrier

- Decreases production of mucin and secretory IgA, antimicrobials that protect your gut

- Promotes overgrowth of opportunistic bacteria like E. coli and Clostridium

- Impairs glucose metabolism and tissue regeneration pathways

- Disrupts circadian rhythm signaling between your gut microbiota and circadian genes

Experts recommend adults get 7-9 hours of quality sleep each night for optimal gut health and microbiome diversity. Here are some tips for improving sleep:

- Keep a consistent bedtime and wake time to reinforce circadian rhythms

- Avoid screen time for 1-2 hours before bedtime

- Create an ideal relaxing sleep environment that is cooler, darker and distraction-free

- Follow a soothing pre-bedtime routine like taking a bath, gentle yoga, reading, etc.

- Take magnesium, glycine, chamomile tea or other natural sleep aids

- Use blackout curtains, sleep mask, ear plugs or a white noise machine if needed

- Deal with stress through earlier meditation, journaling or breathing exercises

Optimizing your sleep quality and duration gives your intestinal tissues the rejuvenation time they need for proper repair and immune protection. Make sufficient high-quality sleep a top priority for maintaining long-term gut wellness.

Gut-Supporting Exercises

Certain types of exercise are very beneficial for supporting healthy gut function, while intense exercises like marathon running can sometimes irritate an already inflamed or compromised GI system.

Gentle, restorative exercise provides these advantages for your gut health:

- Stimulates motility and shortens intestinal transit time to alleviate constipation

- Increases blood flow to GI tissues to deliver oxygen and nutrients

- Reduces inflammation by raising body temperature and increasing circulation

- Promotes development of new blood vessels in the intestines to aid tissue repair

- Triggers an anti-inflammatory environment via release of muscle-produced cytokines

- Regulates glucose metabolism and insulin sensitivity

- Increases production of stress-relieving endorphins

Aim for 30-60 minutes of gut-friendly exercise 4-6 days per week. Here are some excellent gut-supporting workouts:

- Yoga – Gentle flowing or restorative yoga poses massage your internal organs.

- Pilates – Controlled movements strengthen core and aid circulation.

- Walking – Low to moderate pace walking stimulates motility.

- Tai chi – Slow flowing motions combined with deep breathing relax the body.

- Swimming – Low-impact laps gently stimulate the intestines.

- Rowing – Rhythmic rowing motions massage the GI tract.

- Qigong – Flowing sequences harmonize breath, movement and imagery.

- Dancing – Graceful, free-form dance moves gently stretch and bend the torso.

While exercise reduces GI inflammation and supports healthy motility, be cautious exercising intensely with a compromised gut, as the exertion and jostling could further irritate an already disturbed intestinal lining. Prioritize gentle activities that relax the body over high-intensity workouts. Move your body daily in ways that feel healing.

Sustaining Microbiome Diversity Long-Term

Now that your gut is healed, it's crucial to maintain the diversity and balance of your gut microbiota to support lifelong optimal function. Here are some tips:

- Continue eating fermented foods like yogurt, kefir, kimchi, etc. that provide live probiotics. Rotate through different types for variety.

- Take spore-based probiotic supplements like Megasporebiotic that powerfully colonize your intestines with beneficial bacteria.

- Include prebiotic fibers in your meals daily such as garlic, onion, asparagus, apples, flaxseed, chia seeds etc. to nourish probiotics.

- Stay hydrated with filtered water, herbal teas, bone broth and fresh vegetable juices to support elimination.

- Consider periodic cleansing protocols such as bone broth fasts, juice fasts or digestive system resets to give your GI tract a rest.

- Avoid unnecessary antibiotics which deplete your microbiome. Only use them for diagnosed infections, and always follow with probiotic foods and supplements.

- Address any low stomach acid, pancreatic insufficiency or other digestive impairments limiting your ability to break down prebiotics.

- Check for hidden sources of food sensitivities like gluten, dairy or soy lurking in packaged goods. Read labels.

- Keep refined sugar and artificial sweetener intake low, as these compromise the microbiome.

- Limit use of NSAIDs, antacids, steroids or other medications that can alter gut flora.

- Reduce toxin exposure from processed foods, chemicals in personal care and home products, unfiltered water, etc.

Making long-term gut-protective lifestyle choices allows you to sustain the gains you've achieved through your leaky gut healing journey. With diligence, you can maintain a diverse, thriving microbiome and healthy intestinal barrier for life!

Key Takeaways:

Optimizing certain lifestyle factors outside of nutrition provides immense gut-healing benefits:

- Managing stress daily through activities like meditation, yoga, and time in nature counteracts inflammation.

- Prioritizing 7-9 hours of quality sleep nightly allows intestinal tissues to regenerate.

- Engaging in gentle, relaxing exercise like walking, Pilates, tai chi supports motility.

- Continuing fermented foods, periodic cleansing, avoiding gut-disrupting medications preserves microbial diversity.

By protecting your microbiome, soothing your digestive system, providing ample down-time for tissue repair, and avoiding sources of irritation; you solidify your gut healing wins for the long term. With dedication to healthy lifestyle practices, you can maintain optimal gut function fr life!

Conclusion

If you've made it to this point in the book, congratulations! You now have a comprehensive understanding of how to heal leaky gut syndrome and cultivate a healthy gut microbiome with the power of whole foods and strategic lifestyle practices.

In this conclusion chapter, we'll recap the key components from your 4-week gut healing journey. You'll come away with a solid action plan for restoring optimal digestive health from the inside out. Let's explore the main steps:

Step 1: Remove Gut Irritants

The first step on the path to healing leaky gut is removing inflammatory foods, gut irritants, and anything else that compromises your intestinal lining. As covered in Chapter 2, these dietary eliminations are essential during Week 1 of your gut healing protocol:

- Gluten, dairy, corn, soy, eggs, nightshades and any personal food sensitivities

- Refined sugars and excess carbs that feed opportunistic bacteria and yeast

- Factory-farmed meat which contains antibiotics and stress hormones

- Fried foods, alcohol, coffee, artificial additives which are hard on your GI tract

- Any medications known to disrupt healthy gut flora and stomach acid levels

Removing these inflammatory compounds gives your GI tract a chance to calm inflammation and reset. Be diligent, as even small traces of irritants can perpetuate leaky gut in those with compromised intestinal lining integrity.

Step 2: Replace with Gut Soothers

After removing irritants, week 2 of your gut healing plan involves replacing those inflammatory foods with ingredients proven to soothe, heal and seal a damaged gut lining. Emphasize these gut nourishing superfoods:

- Bone broth, cooked from scratch to extract gut-soothing amino acids like glycine

- Wild caught fish like salmon and mackerel containing anti-inflammatory omega-3 fats

- Pastured eggs with 18 amino acids to nourish intestinal tissue

- Fermented foods like kimchi, kefir, sauerkraut and yogurt containing probiotics

- Prebiotic fiber from onions, garlic, bananas, apples, dandelion greens and nuts

- Anti-inflammatory fats like olive oil, avocado, ghee and coconut

- Soothing herbal teas like marshmallow root, licorice, slippery elm and ginger

- Collagen peptides, L-glutamine and aloe vera supplements to heal leaky gut

Replacing with these nourishing foods and supplements helps provide your body the building blocks it needs to begin repairing your intestinal barrier during week 2.

Step 3: Reinoculate with Beneficial Bacteria

Restoring balance in your gut microbiome is a pivotal piece of the gut healing puzzle. Week 3 emphasizes strategic ways to reinoculate your ecosystem with beneficial strains of bacteria.

- Take a high quality, high potency probiotic supplement with diverse bacterial strains

- Consume traditionally fermented foods like kimchi and kefir that contain live cultures

- Drink bone broth, which acts as a prebiotic to nourish probiotics

- Eat prebiotic fibers like garlic, onion, dandelion greens and leeks

- Consider spore-based probiotics that colonize deep in your intestines

- Avoid unnecessary antibiotics which kill off your microbiome

Reinoculating helpful bacteria trains your immune system not to overreact and strengthens the intestinal barrier against future pathogens.

Step 4: Repair and Reinforce the Gut Lining

The final phase of your gut healing journey focuses on sealing up the loose junctions between intestinal cells and reinforcing your gut barrier using key supplements:

- L-glutamine to regenerate enterocytes and tighten cell junctions

- Zinc carnosine to heal gut lining and reduce inflammation

- Aloe vera to soothe inflammation and decrease permeability

- Slippery elm to coat and protect your GI tract

- Marshmallow root to stimulate healing mucus production

- Butyrate to nourish colon cells and strengthen tight junctions

- DGL licorice to combat leaky gut induced inflammation

Repairing and sealing your intestinal lining prevents future leakage of undigested particles into your bloodstream where they trigger inflammation.

Step 5: Support with Gut-Healing Lifestyle Factors

In addition to removing irritants, replacing with gut soothers, reinoculating microbiome diversity, and repairing your intestinal barrier, certain lifestyle factors covered in Chapter 4 help solidify your gut healing wins:

- Managing daily stress through techniques like meditation, breathwork, yoga, nature time, and float therapy. Chronic stress damages gut lining integrity.

- Getting 7-9 hours of quality sleep nightly. Your intestines regenerate best during overnight deep sleep cycles.

- Engaging in gentle exercise like walking, Pilates, tai chi, swimming and dancing to support motility and circulation.

- Continuing fermented foods, periodic cleansing, and avoiding medications that disrupt your microbiome diversity.

Optimizing these key lifestyle pillars provides immense gut-balancing benefits synergistic with your dietary protocols.

Step 6: Stay Diligent About Avoiding Triggers

Once your leaky gut is healed, it's important not to undo your progress. Continue avoiding inflammatory and highly reactive foods that compromise your intestinal lining like gluten, conventional dairy, factory farmed animals, fried foods, alcohol and artificial additives. Read labels diligently and know how to spot hidden sources of food sensitivities when grocery shopping and eating out.

You may also wish to continue eliminating grains, legumes, eggs, nightshades, nuts, seeds and high FODMAP fruits and vegetables for a time if you have autoimmunity or lingering food sensitivities. Check food reintroductions carefully for symptoms.

Stay disciplined about steering clear of gut irritants and enjoys the lifelong benefits of a healthy intestinal barrier and thriving inner ecosystem!

Gut Healing Recipes and Meal Planning

Chapter 3 of this book provided 50 delicious gut-healing recipes to include in your leaky gut protocol and beyond. Refer back to those recipes for anti-inflammatory breakfasts, salads, main dishes, snacks, probiotic foods and drinks, herbal elixirs and more.

Continue emphasizing similar whole food recipes centered around ingredients that heal and seal the gut lining like bone broth, collagen, sauerkraut, aloe, herbs, and healthy fats. Avoid inflammatory triggers. Meal prep batches of gut-friendly foods like soups, smoothies, and snacks for grab-and-go convenience.

Let these recipes guide you as you continues to nourish your microbiome with every meal. Share them with friends and family to spread the gut healing wisdom!

Troubleshooting Setbacks and Symptoms

It's normal to hit some bumps in the road on your gut healing journey. You may experience die-off symptoms like headache, fatigue, rashes, or nausea as pathogenic bacteria and biofilms release toxins. This is a sign your protocols are working! Stay hydrated, reduce detox supports like binders, and wait it out.

If you indulge in a food sensitivity or suffer a major stress, don't beat yourself up. Just get back on track with your gut-healing protocols. Patience and consistency are key. It takes time to reverse long-standing intestinal permeability and microbial imbalances. Trust the process!

Customizing Your Long-Term Gut Healing Plan

You now have a comprehensive blueprint for overcoming leaky gut syndrome using the power of food as medicine and strategic lifestyle changes. As you continue applying these protocols, keep customizing your plan based on your unique situation, symptoms and food tolerances.

Experiment with elimination diets like Paleo AIP if you have autoimmunity. Try low FODMAP if IBS is an issue. Rotate food reintroductions cautiously. Note symptom triggers. Work with a functional nutritionist if needed for personalized testing and guidance.

Keep emphasizing gut superfoods, microbial diversity, stress relief, rest, gentle movement, and hydration. Fine tune your long-term gut nourishing lifestyle so you can feel your absolute best every day!

The Future of Gut and Microbiome Health

This is just the beginning of our understanding of the immense role our gut flora and intestinal barrier play in whole body health and disease prevention. There are trillions of bacteria in the human microbiome, most of which we have yet to isolate and study. Personalized microbiome analysis will continue illuminating the connections between specific strains of bacteria and various health conditions.

Exciting microbiome research is underway exploring:

- Direct links between gut flora and mental health disorders like depression and anxiety

- How an infant's early life microbiome impacts lifelong neurological development

- Using fecal microbial transplants to treat autoimmunity and other diseases by resetting gut flora

- Prebiotic foods, herbs and supplements to help colonize beneficial bacteria

- Probiotic strains to target digestion, immunity, cognition, metabolism and hormones

- The ability of a healthy microbiome to offset risks for obesity, diabetes and heart disease

- Microbiome-based diagnostics predicting risk for specific cancers

The gut-brain axis is proving to be one of the most fascinating frontiers in gut health, with clear pathways between your intestinal flora, enteric nervous system and brain. We have much more to learn about how cultivating a thriving inner garden translates to lifelong physical and mental thriving.

In many ways, healing leaky gut and imbalances in your microbiome gives you a "clean slate" upon which optimal whole body wellness can flourish. Everything is interconnected. When we nourish our microbiome, reduce inflammation, and heal our gut, we provide the fertile soil from which our very best health can blossom.

My hope is that through reading this book, you feel empowered and equipped with the scientific understanding and practical dietary and lifestyle tools needed to transform your gut health and therefore, your whole quality of life. Are you ready to continue your exciting gut healing journey? Let's begin planting the seeds for your newfound wellness starting today!

Additional Resources

To take your education on gut health to the next level, check out these recommended resources:

Podcasts:

- The Gut Healing Podcast by Jordan Reasoner and Steve Wright

- Revolution Health Radio by Chris Kresser

- The Doctor's Farmacy by Dr. Mark Hyman

Books:

- The Gut Healing Protocol by John Herron

- Healthy Gut, Healthy You by Michael Ruscio

- The Microbiome Diet by Raphael Kellman

- The Cleansing Program by Dr. Alejandro Junger

Documentaries:

- Gut by Cambria Glosz

- Microcosmos

- The Microbiome - A Secret World Inside You

Functional Nutritionists:

- Kalish Institute

- Functional Medicine Coaching Academy

- Nutritional Therapy Association

Testing:

- GI Map by Diagnostic Solutions

- Organic Acids Test by Great Plains Lab

- Viome Gut Microbiome Analysis

Supplements:

- Megasporebiotic spore probiotics

- Apex Energetics GI Restore Powder

- Pure Encapsulations Zinc Carnosine

- Designs for Health GI Revive Powder

Final Encouragement

While healing your gut takes commitment, patience, and trial and error, it is absolutely possible and so very worth it. I hope the detailed guidance in this book empowers you to take control of your health starting with your gut.

Remember to show compassion towards yourself on tougher days. Celebrate each small win. Stay focused on the incredible benefits you'll experience by nourishing your microbiome and sealing your leaky gut for good. The future of whole body wellness starts here! Now go cultivate the thriving garden within you. Wishing you profound gut health and happiness!

Printed in Dunstable, United Kingdom